SALAD COOKBOOK 2022

DELICIOUS RECIPES TO BE HEALTHIER

PAUL PAIRE

Table of Contents

Creamy crunchy slaw

Ingredients

A cup of mayonnaise

2 tbsp. Cider vinegar

1 tsp. Caraway seeds

1 head Cabbages, shredded

2 Scallions, chopped

2 Green apples, cut into slices

1 cup Bacon

Salt and pepper, to taste

Method

The mayonnaise is to be mixed it the caraway seeds and the cider vinegar. When mixed properly, toss the mixture with the finely chopped cabbages, scallion, green apples and cooked bacons. Now mix the ingredients well, and then season to taste, if required add salt and pepper, to taste and then keep aside for a while before serving.

Enjoy!!

Bistro bacon salad

Ingredients

1 cup Bacon

2 tbsp. Cider vinegar

1 tsp. Dijon mustard

Olive oil

1 bunch mesclun greens

Salt and pepper, to taste

1 Egg, poached

Method

The bacons are to be fried at first and then the fried bacons are to be chopped. Now mix the cider vinegar, Dijon mustard, olive oil, salt and pepper in a bowl. After mixing all these ingredients properly, toss this mixture with the mesclun greens. Then top the salad with the chopped bacons and poached egg.

Enjoy!!

Curried tuna salad

Ingredients

1 tsp. Curry powder

Vegetable oil

½ cup A cup of mayonnaise

Lime juice

A can of tuna

2 Red onions, cut into slices

1 bunch Cilantro

10-12 Golden raisins

Salt and pepper, to taste

Method

The curry powder is to be toasted in the vegetable oil and then keep it aside to cool. Now take the mayonnaise, lime juice, salt and pepper to a bowl and mix them well. Now take the toasted powder and this mixture and toss it with the canned tune, cilantro, red onions and raisin. Mix them well and then serve the delicious to taste, interesting salad.

Enjoy!!

Cranberry spinach salad

Ingredients

½ cup Butter

Less than a cup of almonds, blanched

A pound of spinach, chopped in pieces

A cup of cranberries, dried

1 tsp. Sesame seeds, toasted

1 tsp. Poppy seeds

1/2 a cup of white sugar

1 Onion, minced

1 tsp. Paprika

About 1/2 a cup of white wine vinegar

Cider vinegar

1/2 a cup of vegetable oil

Method

Take a pan and melt the butter in it in the oil over a low heat and then mix the almonds in it and toast it. And when toasted, let it cool for a while. Now take another medium sized bowl, mix the sesame seeds, poppy seeds, sugar, onion, with the white wine vinegar, cider vinegar and the oil. Then mix this mixture with the spinach and finally toss it in the bowl of toasted almonds and the dried cranberries. Then the salad is ready to be served.

Enjoy!!

Bermuda spinach salad

Ingredients

5-6 Eggs

1/2 a pound of bacon

About two pounds of spinach, finely chopped

3 Croutons

1 cup Mushrooms

1 Onion

A cup of white sugar

Vegetable oil

1 tsp. Black pepper, ground

Celery seeds

1 tsp. Dijon mustard

Method

Take the eggs to a pan and cover the pan wholly with cold water and then bring the water to boil, and then let the egg settle in the water, so keep the pan aside and cool it. When the eggs are cool, peel and chop them. Now take the bacons to a pan and cook it until brown in color. After cooking them, drain it. Now take the rest of the ingredients and mix it well. When mixed well, the salad is ready to be served.

Enjoy!!

Spinach and mushroom salad

Ingredients

1 pound Bacon, cut into slices

3 Eggs

1 tsp. White sugar

2-3 tbsp. of water

2 tbsp. of cider vinegar

A pound of spinach

Salt

About a pound of mushrooms, cut in slices

Method

Take a large sized pan, and cook the slices of bacon in oil over a medium heat. When the bacons turn its color to brown, crumble it and set it aside and at the same time the bacon fat is to be reserved. Now take the eggs to the pan and cover in with water and then bring the water to boil. After take the eggs out and cool, then peel and cut the eggs in wedges. Now take the sugar, water, vinegar and salt to the pan with the bacon fat and heat them thoroughly. Now take all the ingredients with the spinach to a large sized bowl, mixed them and thus the delicious salad is ready to be served.

Enjoy!!

Wilted Spinach Salad

Ingredients

3 Eggs

A pound of bacon, sliced

Bunch of spinach, cleaned and dried

About a cup of sugar

1/2 a cup of white vinegar

A cup of red wine vinegar

3 Green onions

Method

Take the eggs to a pan and cover them with sufficient cold water and then bring the water to boil, by covering the pan. When the eggs are done, set in aside to cool and then peel and cut the eggs in slices or wedges. Now take the bacons to the pan and cook them over a low heat. When the bacons are browned in color, transfer them to a large sized bowl with the spinach and green onions. Pour the bacon fat and the rest of the ingredients to the bowl, mix well and then the salad is ready to be served.

Enjoy!!

Warm Brussels Sprouts, Bacon and spinach salad

Ingredients

6-7 Bacon slices

2 cups of Brussels sprouts

1 tsp. Caraway seeds

2 tbsp. Vegetable oil

2 tbsp. White wine vinegar

1/2 pound of spinach, chopped, rinsed and dried

Method

The bacon is to be taken to a pan and cooked over a medium heat, until the bacon is browned in color. After it is cooked, crumble and then set them aside. Now the sprouts are to be steamed until they are softened. In the remaining bacon fat of the pan, add the sprouts with the caraway seeds and stir them for a minute or two until they are tendered. Now take all the ingredients along with the bacons, spinach to a bowl and then mix well. When mixed well, the delicious salad is ready to serve.

Enjoy!!

Broccoli Salad

Ingredients

1 cup of low fat mayonnaise

2 Broccoli heads, fresh, cut in pieces

1/2 cup of red onions, finely chopped

1/2 cup of raisin

2 tbsp. White wine vinegar

1 tsp. White sugar1 cup of sunflower seeds

Method

Take the bacons to a pan and cook them over medium heat, until they are browned. Then drain the bacons and keep it at a side. Now take all the ingredients to a bowl, along with the cooked bacon and mix them well. When they are mixed, refrigerate it for an hour or two and then serve it chilled.

Enjoy!!

Harvest Salad

Ingredients

1/2 cup of walnuts, chopped

1 bunch of spinach, cleaned and torn in bites

1/2 a cup of cranberries

1/2 cup of blue cheese, shredded or crumbled

2 Tomatoes, deseeded and chopped

1 avocado, peeled and cut in dice

2 tbsp. Red wine vinegar

2 tbsp. Red raspberry jam

1 cup of walnut oil

Salt and black pepper, to taste

Method

The oven is to be preheated to 190C and then the walnuts are to be arranged in a baking sheet and are to be then toasted until they are browned. Now take a bowl and mix the spinach, walnuts, cranberries, red onions, avocado, blue cheese and tomatoes. When mixed properly, take another small sized bowl and mix the jam, walnut oil, pepper and salt and the vinegar. Now pour this mixture to the salad and mix them well. Before serving cool it for an hour or two.

Enjoy!!

Winter green salad

Ingredients

1 bunch Collard leaves, chopped

1 bunch of kale leaves, chopped

1 Romaine lettuce, trimmed

1 head of red cabbage

1 pear

1 Bermuda onion

1 Avocado, peeled and diced

2 Carrots, grated

2-3 tbsp. Raisins

Olive oil

Vinegar

1 tsp. Honey

1 tsp. Oregano

1 tsp. Dijon mustard

1 Garlic clove, minced

Peppercorns

Method

Take a large sized bowl and toss the collard leaves, kale, and grated carrots with the cabbage, walnuts, tomatoes and raisins and mix them together. Now take another small bowl and take the rest of the ingredients in it and mix them well. When the ingredients are mixed well, take the mixture and pour it over the bowl of cabbages and collard leaves, and coat them all properly. Thus it is ready to be served.

Enjoy!!

Tomato mozzarella salad

Ingredients

5 Tomatoes

1 cup Mozzarella cheese, cut in slices

2 tbsp. Olive oil

2 tbsp. Balsamic vinegar

Salt and pepper to taste

Fresh leaves of basil, torn in pieces

Method

Take the tomatoes and mozzarellas on a serving dish and place them in an alternate manner. Now the oil, vinegar, salt and the pepper are to be mixed and then are to be poured over the serving dish. Before serving the salad, sprinkle the basil leaves over the salad.

Enjoy!!

BLT salad

Ingredients

1 pound of bacon

1 cup of mayonnaise

1 tsp. Garlic powder

Salt and pepper, to taste

1 head Romaine

2Tomatoes

2 Croutons

Method

The bacons are to be cook in a pan over a medium heat until they are evenly browned in color and then drain them and set at a side. Now take a food processor and process the mayonnaise, milk, garlic powder, pepper, until they are smooth in texture. Thus the dressing of the salad is ready. Now toss the lettuce, cooked bacons, tomatoes and croutons in a bowl and then pour the dressing and coat them properly. Before serving cool it for an hour or two.

Enjoy!!

Beautiful salad

Ingredients

1 bunch Baby spinach leaves

2 Red onions

1 can of mandarin oranges, drained

1 cup Cranberries, dried

½ cup Feta cheese, crumbled

1 cup of vinaigrette salad dressing mix

Method

Take all the ingredients except the salad dressing mix, to a large sized bowl and mix them well. When the ingredients are properly mixed, sprinkle the salad dressing mix over the bowl of salad and thus the beautiful salad is ready to be served.

Enjoy!!

Almond mandarin salad

Ingredients

1/2 pound of bacon

2 tsp. White wine vinegar

1 tsp. Honey

1 tsp. Hot mustard

1 tsp. Celery salt

1 tsp. Paprika

1 Red leaf lettuce

1 can of mandarin oranges, drained

2 Green onions, cut in wedges

1 cup of almond, silvered

Method

Take a pan and cook the bacon, covering them, until they turn brown in color. For preparing the salad dressing, blend the honey, vinegar, mustard with the celery salt, paprika and olive oil. Now the lettuce, oranges, cooked bacons and the silvered almonds are to be tossed in to a bowl and then pour the salad dressing over it and mix them well so that they are well coated. Before serving the salad, let them cool for an hour.

Enjoy!!

Tuna and mandarin salad

Ingredients

Olive oil

1 can of tuna

1 pack of mixed baby greens

1 granny smith apple, peeled and chopped

1 can of mandarin oranges

Method

The olive oil is to be heated and the tuna is to be sautéed until cooked completely. Now take a bowl and toss the salad greens with the sautéed tuna, apples and the oranges. Thus, the salad is ready to be served.

Enjoy!!

Macaroni and tuna fish salad

Ingredients

1 packet of macaroni

2 cans of tuna

1 cup mayonnaise

Salt and pepper, to taste

1 pinch Garlic powder

1 pinch of oregano, dried

1 Onion, finely shredded

Method

Take salted water to a pot and bring it to boil and then add the macaroni and cook them, after cooking them drain the macaroni and then cool it. Now the cans of tuna are to be mixed with the cooked macaroni and then add the mayonnaise to it and mix them well. Now add the rest of the ingredients to the mixture and mix them well. When all the ingredients are mixed, let them cool for about an hour or two. Thus the delicious tuna fish salad is ready to be served.

Enjoy!!

Asian salad

Ingredients

2 pack of ramen noodles

1 cup of almonds, blanched and silvered

2 tsp. Sesame seeds

1/2 cup of butter

1 head of Napa cabbage, chopped

1 bunch of green onions, chopped

¼ cup Vegetable oil

2-3 tsp. White sugar

2 tsp. Soy sauce

Method

Take a pan and heat the butter or margarine and then pour the ramen noodles, sesame seeds and almonds in it over low heat and cook them, until they are browned. When cooked, let them cool. Now take a small sized pan and pour the vegetable oil, sugar and vinegar and then bring them to boil for about a minute and then cool it and when cooled, add the soy sauce in it. Take a bowl and then mix all the ingredients along with the cooked ramen noodles and the sugar mixture and then toss them well. Before serving the salad, let it cool for an hour or more.

Enjoy!!

Asian chicken pasta salad

Ingredients

1 packet Rotelle pasta

2 Chicken breasts, boneless, cut in pieces, cooked

2-3 tbsp. Vegetable oil

Salt

2-3 carrots, shredded

1/2 pound of mushrooms

1/2 head of broccoli

1/2 head of cauliflower

Water

2 tsp. Soy sauce

2 tsp. Sesame oil

Method

Take salted water in a pot and bring it to boil, now add the pack of pasta in it and cook them. When cooked, drain the pasta and set aside. Now take a pan and cook the carrots with salt until they are crispy and tender. Now take a bowl and add the pasta, carrots with chicken breasts and mix them well. Now cook the mushrooms and take it to the bowl and then add the rest of the ingredients to it and mix well. Serve the salad chilled.

Enjoy!!

Cobb salad

Ingredients

4-5 Bacon slices2 Eggs

1 head Iceberg lettuce

1 Chicken breast

2 Tomatoes, sliced

¼ cup Blue cheese, shredded

2 Green onions, sliced

A bottle of salad dressing

Method

Boil the eggs, peel and chop. Pan fry the bacon and chicken, separately until browned. Crumble. Just before serving, combine all the ingredients in a large mixing bowl and mix well. Serve without delay.

Enjoy!!

Arugula Corn Salad with Bacon Recipe

Ingredients

4 large corns

2 cups of chopped arugula

4 strips of bacon

1/3 cup of chopped green onions

1 tbsp. olive oil

1 tbsp. wine vinegar

1/8 tsp. cumin

Salt and black pepper

Method

Heat the corn, in their husks, also on the grill for a smoky flavor, for 12-15 minutes. In a medium sized basin, combine the corn, arugula, bacon, and onions. In a separate basin, beat the vinegar, oil, salt and pepper. Mix covering into salad just before serving and serve without delay.

Enjoy!

Black Eyed Pea Salad Recipe

Ingredients

2 cups of dry black-eyed peas

230grams feta cheese

230grams of sun-dried tomatoes

1 cup Kalamata black olives

Finely chopped green onion

Chopped garlic clove

1 large bunch of chopped spinach

Juice and Zest of a lemon

Method

Cook the peas in salinated water until just done. Drain and wash with cold water. In a bowl mix all the ingredients except for the lemon juice. Add the lemon juice just before serving and serve immediately.

Enjoy!

Arugula Salad with Beets and Goat Cheese Recipe

Ingredients

Salad Ingredients:

2 Peeled Beets

Handful of Arugula leaves

½ cup Goat cheese, crumbled

½ cup Walnuts, chopped

Dressing Ingredients:

¼ cup Olive oil

½ Lemon

¼ tsp. Dry powdered mustard

¾ tsp. Sugar

Salt and pepper

Method

For the dressing combine together the ¼ tsp. of powdered mustard, ¾ tsp. of sugar, ½ lemon, and ¼ cup of olive oil, salt and pepper to flavor. Combine a handful of arugula leaves, a few beet juliennes, crumbled goat cheese and chopped walnuts. Top with the dressing just before serving. Serve without delay.

Enjoy!

Asian Coleslaw Recipe

Ingredients

1 cup Creamy peanut butter

6 tbsp. vegetable oil

½ tsp. toasted sesame oil

4 tbsp. seasoned rice vinegar

4 cups of thinly sliced cabbage

½ cup grated carrots

¼ cup toasted peeled peanuts

Method

Add peanut butter in an average basin and add the toasted sesame oil and beat until nicely softly. Toast the peanuts to get even better flavor with just a minute toasting. Transfer peanuts from pan to a huge bowl. Toss the carrots, cabbage and peanuts together, and any other ingredients you care to add and Serve without delay.

Enjoy!

Asian Noodle Salad Recipe

Ingredients

280grams Chinese noodles

1/3 cup soy sauce

3 cups of broccoli florets

115 grams green gram bean sprouts

3 thinly sliced onions,

1 red bell pepper

1/4 thinly sliced bulky cabbage

1 huge peeled carrot

Method

Pour 4 glasses of water into huge pot, add Chinese noodles. Mix the noodles constantly while they cook. Ensure you follow the noodle package instructions, if using Chinese noodles, they should be done after 5minutes of cooking. Drain noodles, wash with cold water to stop the cooking, extend the noodles out on a sheet pan to air dry. Add broccoli florets and sufficient water to come up to the level of the steamer. Cover and steam cook for 4 minutes. Combine all the ingredients in a bowl. Serve without delay.

Enjoy!

Asparagus Artichoke Salad Recipe

Ingredients

1 large thinly sliced onion

3 tbsp. lemon juice

450grams thick asparagus

2 tbsp. olive oil

1 tsp. garlic powder

1 pint grape

Method

First immerse the sliced onions in the lemon juice, and roast the asparagus in a preheated oven at 400 degrees F. For the asparagus spears add 1 tbsp. of olive oil, and salt them well. Place in a single layer in a foil-lined roasting saucepan and cook for 10 minutes until lightly browned. To grill the asparagus, organize your charcoal grill at high temperature, between 5 to 10 minutes. Remove the asparagus from the grill and cut into bite pieces, set the asparagus and all ingredients into a huge bowl and blend to combine and Serve without delay.

Enjoy!

Asparagus Salad with Shrimp Recipe

Ingredients

450grams asparagus

226grams pink salad shrimp

¼ cup of extra-virgin olive oil

1 minced garlic clove

1 tbsp. lemon juice

1 tbsp. minced parsley

Salt and black pepper

Method

Bring an average pot of water to a boil. Add the asparagus to the boiling water and boil for 3 minutes. If they are pre-cooked, remove after 30 seconds. If the shrimps are raw, boil them for 3 minutes, until cooked through. Remove the shrimp and add them to a huge bowl. Slice the asparagus spears finely diagonally. Slash the asparagus tips off in one piece. Add the remaining ingredients and toss to combine. Add salt and black pepper to taste. Add more lemon juice if desired, to taste and Serve without delay.

Enjoy!

Blueberry Peach Fruit Salad with Thyme Recipe

Ingredients

4 peaches

4 nectarines

1 cup of blueberries

2 tsp. of chopped thyme fresh

1 tsp. of ginger, grated

¼ cup of lemon juice

1 tsp. of lemon zest

1/2 cup of water

¼ cup of sugar

Method

Place the water and sugar into a saucepot and heat to a simmer and cook liquid is reduced by half into simple syrup, allow to cool. Chop up the nectarines and peaches and Add them in a basin with the blueberries. Pour over the cooled syrup. Add the lemon zest, thyme, lemon juice, and ginger. Blend and cover up with plastic wrap, place in the refrigerator and allow macerating for one hour. Serve without delay.

Enjoy!

Broccoli Salad Recipe

Ingredients

salt

6 cups broccoli florets

1/2 cup of toasted almonds

1/2 cup cooked bacon

¼ cup of chopped onion

1 cup of thawed frozen peas

1 cup of mayonnaise

apple cider vinegar

¼ cup of honey

Method

Bring a huge pot of water, salted with a tsp. of salt, to a simmer. Add the broccoli florets. Cook 2 minutes, depending on how crispy you want the broccoli. 1 minute will turn the broccoli bright greenish color, and leave it still pretty crispy. Set your regulator and do not cook for more than 2 minutes. Combine broccoli florets, crumbled bacon, almonds, chopped onion, and peas in a huge serving basin in a separate pudding basin, beat together mayonnaise, vinegar and honey and flip to blend well, Chill thoroughly before. Serve without delay.

Enjoy!

Broccoli Slaw with Cranberry Orange Dressing Recipe

Ingredients

2 tbsp. balsamic vinegar

½ cup dried sweetened cranberries

2 tsp. whole grain mustard

2 tbsp. red wine vinegar

1 clove garlic

½ cup orange juice

2-3 slices orange zest

Kosher salt

6 tbsp. vegetable oil

¼ cup of mayonnaise

½ head cabbage

2-3 green onions

¼ cup dried cranberries

2-3 slices grated orange zest

Method

Add the red wine vinegar and balsamic vinegar, mustard, plumped dried cranberries, honey, garlic, orange juice, orange zest, and salt into a food processor and pulsate until pureed soft. Gradually add the vegetable oil, while blending, to form a good mixture. Then add the mayonnaise and pulse until combined. Add grated broccoli stalks, carrots, dried cranberries, orange zest, and kosher salt into a mixing bowl. Add the dressing and toss to combine, until the dressing is evenly distributed. Serve without delay.

Enjoy!

Avocado Salad with Heirloom Tomatoes

Ingredients

1 1/2 sliced and peeled avocados

1 1/2 tomatoes, sliced

2 Sliced green onions or chopped fresh chives

Lemon Juice from one slice

A pinch of coarse salt

Method

Arrange slices of avocado and tomato on a plate. Drizzle lemon juice over chives, and coarse salt. Remove the pit from one half of an avocado still in its skin, and remove its pulp in a bowl. Add in the tomato and prepared chives and mix well. Serve without delay.

Enjoy!

Cardamom Citrus Fruit Salad Recipe

Ingredients

1 huge ruby pink grapefruit

3 combination of navel oranges or navel oranges or mandarin orange, blood oranges and or tangerines

¼ cup of honey

2 tbsp. fresh lemon or lime juice

1/4 tsp. of ground cardamom

Method

First unpeel the fruit, cut away the membranes of the segments with a sharp knife. Bring together the peeled segments in an addition bowl. Conduit off any surplus juice from the fruit into diminutive saucepan. Add the honey, lime juice and cardamom to the saucepan. Boil for 10 minutes and then remove from heat and let chill to room temperature. Let stand for 15 minutes or put on ice until ready. Serve without delay.

Enjoy!

Capers Corn Salad Recipe

Ingredients

6 ears of sweet corn

¼ cup of olive oil

sherry vinegar

black pepper

1 ½ tsp. kosher salt

½ tsp. sugar

3 chopped seeded tomatoes

½ cup sliced scallions

230grams fresh mozzarella

basil leaves

Method

Arrange your grill on high heat, and place the corn cobs in their husks directly on the grill. Cook for 15 minutes, there is no need to immerse the corn in water first if the corn is fresh. If you want some burn on the corn itself, remove a few of the outer corn husks first, so there is less of a caring layer around the corn. Take a huge bowl, and flip together the corn, Mozzarella, scallions, tomatoes, and the dressing. Right before serving, stir in the freshly sliced basil. Serve without delay.

Enjoy!

Celery Root Salad

Ingredients

½ cup mayonnaise

2 tbsp. mustard, Dijon

1 tbsp. lemon juice

2 tbsp. parsley, chopped

545gm celery root equally quartered, peeled & coarsely grated just before mixing

½ tart green apple, peeled, cored, julienned

Salt and ground pepper

Method

Combine mayonnaise with mustard along with lemon juice and parsley in a bowl. Crinkle celery root with apple and season with salt & pepper, wrap it up and refrigerate until cooled, 1 hour.

Enjoy!

Cherry Tomato Cucumber Feta Salad

Ingredients

2 or 3 cups of cherry tomatoes, sliced into two halves

1 cup chopped cucumber, peeled

1/4 cup crumbled cheese, feta

1 tbsp. mint chiffonaded leaves

1 tbsp. oregano, fresh, chopped

1 tbsp. lemon juice

2 tbsp. shallots or green onions, finely chopped

2 tbsp. olive oil

Salt

Method

Softly toss the cherry tomatoes along with cucumber, cheese, onions, mint & oregano together. Garnish with lemon juice and salt & pepper along with olive oil.

Enjoy!

Cucumber Salad with Mint and Feta Recipe

Ingredients

453 grams cucumbers, thinly sliced

¼ thinly sliced red onion, and cut into 1-inch extensive segments

2 - 3 thinly sliced red radishes

10 thinly sliced mint leaves

White vinegar

Olive oil

¼ of pound feta cheese

freshly ground pepper and Salt

Method

In an average sized mixing bowl, smoothly mix the sliced cucumbers, mint leaves, radishes, red onion with a diminutive bit of white vinegar and olive oil, salt and freshly ground pepper to flavor. Just before serving, shake over on crumbled bits of feta cheese. Serve immediately before any delay.

Enjoy!

Cherry Tomato Orzo Salad Recipe

Ingredients

230 grams orzo pasta

Salt and Black pepper to taste

1 pint sliced in half red cherry tomatoes

1 pint sliced in half yellow cherry tomatoes

¼ cup of olive oil

230 grams crumbled feta cheese

1 huge chopped and peeled cucumber

2 green thinly sliced onions

fresh minced oregano

Method

Fill a big pot with water and bring to a boil. Add the orzo, stirring it so that it doesn't stick to the bottom of the pan. Cook, at a high boil until al dente, ripe through, but still a bit resolute. Mix with the rest of the ingredients, the tomatoes, oregano, feta cheese, green onions, cucumber and black pepper. Serve without delay.

Enjoy!

Cucumber Salad with Grapes and Almonds Recipe

Ingredients

¼ cup slivered almonds

1 pound peeled cucumbers

salt

1 tsp. garlic, minced

20 sliced green grapes

2 tbsp. olive oil

1 sherry or white wine vinegar

2 tsp. minced chives, for garnish

Method

Slice the cucumbers lengthwise. Use a spoon to scoop out the seeds in the middle, discard the seeds. If using slightly big cucumbers, sliver them again lengthwise. Mix around to coat the salt evenly on the cucumber. Toast the sliced almonds in a small pan on simmering heat, flipping them often, remove in a bowl to cool. Mix the almonds, cucumbers, grapes, garlic, olive oil, and vinegar together in a big bowl and add more salt to taste. Garnish with chives and serve without delay.

Enjoy!

Cucumber Mint Quinoa Salad Recipe

Ingredients

1 cup quinoa

2 cups of water

½ tsp. kosher salt

1 large peeled cucumber

¼ cup thinly sliced mint

1 thinly sliced green onion

4 tbsp. rice vinegar

olive oil

1 peeled avocado

Method

Place the quinoa in a medium sized saucepan, pour in water. Add half a tsp. of salt, diminish to a low heat. Let the cooked quinoa cool to room temperature. You can cool down the quinoa speedily by spreading it out on a sheet pan. Cut the cucumber in long slices. Shake over with seasoned rice vinegar and flip again. Smoothly fold in chop up avocado if using and serve without delay.

Enjoy!

Couscous with Pistachios and Apricots Recipe

Ingredients

½ cup chopped red onion

¼ cup lemon juice

1 box of couscous

2 tbsp. olive oil

½ cup raw pistachios

10 dried chopped apricots

1/3 cup chopped parsley

Method

Put the chopped onion in a little bowl. Empty the lemon juice over the onions set aside and let the onions soak in the lemon juice. Toast the pistachios in a tiny pan on simmering heat until they brown. Put 2 cups of water in a medium saucepan and bring to a boil. Add a tbsp. of olive oil and one tsp. of salt to the water; add the couscous and cook covered for 5-6 minutes. Stir in the pistachios, chopped apricots and parsley. Mix in the red onion and lemon juice. Serve without delay.

Enjoy!

Coleslaw Recipe

Ingredients

½ Cabbage, sliced

½ Carrot, sliced

2 – 3 Green onions, sliced

3 tbsp. Mayonnaise

½ tsp. Yellow mustard

2 tbsp. Rice vinegar

Sugar, to taste

Salt and pepper, to taste

Method

Combine all the sliced vegetables in a bowl. To make the dressing, mix together the mayonnaise, yellow mustard and rice vinegar. Just before serving, drizzle the dressing on the veggies and sprinkle with some salt, pepper and sugar. Serve without delay.

Enjoy!

Cold Pea Salad Recipe

Ingredients

453 grams frozen petite peas, do not thaw

170 grams smokehouse almonds, chopped, rinsed to take off the excess salt, preferably by hand

½ cup of chopped green onions

230 grams chopped water chestnuts

2/3 cup of mayonnaise

2 tbsp. yellow curry powder

Salt to taste

Pepper to taste

Method

Combine the frozen green onions, peas, almonds, and water chestnuts. Combine together the mayonnaise and curry powder in a separate mixing bowl. Smoothly fold the mayonnaise combination into peas. Sprinkle salt and freshly ground black pepper to flavor. Serve without delay.

Enjoy!

Cucumber Yogurt Salad Recipe

Ingredients

2 peeled then sliced cucumbers, quartered lengthwise

1 cup Plain yogurt

1 tsp. a couple of tsps., or dried dill of fresh dill

Salt to taste

Pepper to taste

Method

First taste the cucumbers to make sure that they are not sour. If the cucumber is sour, soak the cucumber slices in salted water for half an hour, or longer, until the bitterness is lost, then rinse and drain before using. To prepare the salad, simply gently combine together the ingredients. Shake over or sprinkle of salt and sprinkle pepper as for flavor. Serve without delay.

Enjoy!

Dad's Greek Salad Recipe

Ingredients

6 tbsp. olive oil

2 tbsp. fresh lemon juice

½ tsp. fresh chopped garlic

4 tablespoons red wine vinegar

½ tsp. dried oregano

½ tsp. dill weed

Salt and freshly ground black pepper

3 bulky seeded plum tomatoes

¾ peeled, coarsely chopped cucumber

½ peeled and chopped red onion

1 bell coarsely chopped pepper

½ cup of chopped pitted black olives

A heaping 1/2 cup crumbled feta cheese

Method

Mix up the vinegar, olive oil, garlic, lemon juice, oregano and dill weed together until blended. Season to taste with salt and freshly ground black pepper. Combine the tomatoes, along with cucumber, onion, bell pepper, olives in a bowl. Sprinkle cheese over and Serve without delay.

Enjoy!

Dad's Potato Salad Recipe

Ingredients

4 peeled midsized Russet potatoes

4 tbsp. juice from kosher dill pickles

3 tbsp. finely chopped dill pickles

¼ cup chopped parsley

½ cup chopped red onion

2 stalks celery

2 chopped scallions

½ cup mayonnaise

2 tsp. Dijon mustard

Kosher salt and ground black pepper to flavor

Method

Put peeled, cut potatoes in a huge pot. Cover with an inch of salted water. Place the pot of water to boil. Simmer for 20 minutes until just fork tender. Remove from pot, let cool until warm. Add celery, parsley, scallions and, the hardboiled egg, carrots, and red bell pepper. Part little basin, blend mayonnaise with mustard. Sprinkle salt and pepper to taste. Serve without delay.

Enjoy!

Endive Salad with Walnuts, Pears, and Gorgonzola Recipe

Ingredients

3 sliced first lengthwise Endive heads, then crosswise in ½ inch slices

2 tbsp. chopped walnuts

2 tbsp. crumbled gorgonzola

1 cored and chopped Bartlett pear,

2 tbsp. olive oil

2 tsp. cider vinegar

Sprinkle of kosher salt and freshly ground black pepper

Method

Put the chopped endive in a huge bowl. Add the crumbled gorgonzola, walnuts, and chopped pears, chop the pears and walnuts more finely. Flip to combine, drizzle olive over the salad with some crumbled blue cheese in the endive leaves, like filling little boats, for appetizers. Sprinkle cider vinegar over the salad. Toss to combine. Season to taste with a shake over of salt and pepper. Serve without delay.

Enjoy!

Fennel Slaw with Mint Vinaigrette Recipe

Ingredients

1 huge fennel bulb

1 ½ tsp. sugar

2 lemon juice

¼ cup olive oil

½ tsp. mustard

½ tsp. salt

1 bunch chopped fresh mint

2 minced shallot

Method

Put together the vinaigrette. Place the lemon juice, onions, salt, mustard, sugar and mint in a mixer and pulse briefly to combine. With the motor running, mix in the olive oil until it is well combined. Using a mandolin, shave the fennel into 1/8 inch piece starting from the bottom of the bulb. Don't worry about coring the fennel bulb, it's preventable. If you don’t have a mandolin, slice the bulb as thin as you can. Cut some of the fennel fronds as well to flip in with the salad. Serve without delay.

Enjoy!

Fennel, Radicchio and Endive Salad Recipe

Ingredients

Salad

1 head radicchio

3 Belgian endives

1 huge fennel bulb

1 cup coarsely grated parmesan cheese

Dressing

3 tbsp. fennel fronds

½ tsp. mustard

3 tsp. minced onion

2 tbsp. lemon juice

1 tsp. salt

1 tsp. sugar

1/3 cup olive oil

Method

Cut the head of radicchio in half, then in quarters. Take each quarter and cut slices of about half inch thick crosswise on the radicchio from the end toward the core. Cut thin slices from each quarter toward the core. Toss all the cut vegetables in a huge bowl with the grated parmesan. Add in the lemon juice, mustard, onion, salt and sugar. Drizzle the olive oil and puree the dressing for 45 second. Serve without delay.

Enjoy!

Festive Beet Citrus Salad with Kale and Pistachios Recipe

Ingredients

10 mix of red beets

3 blood oranges

1 bunch of thinly sliced kale

1 cup roughly chopped roasted pistachios

¼ cup chopped mint leaves

3 chopped Italian parsley

Dressing:

2 tbsp. lemon juice

1/2 cup quality extra virgin olive oil

2 coarsely chopped capers

Salt and pepper to flavor

Method

Cook the beets separately by color. Place each batch of beets in a vessel and cover with about an inch of water. Add in some tsp. of salt. While the beets are cook, organize the dressing. Place all of the dressing ingredients into a container and shake until well mix together. Prepare salad by placing the beets, parsley, over the kale, sprinkling with the chopped roasted pistachios. Serve topped with the prepared dressing.

Enjoy!

Golden Beet and Pomegranate Salad Recipe

Ingredients

3 golden haired beets

1 cup chopped red onion

¼ cup red wine vinegar

¼ cup chicken broth

1 cup of sugar

½ tsp. grated orange peel

¼ cup pomegranate seeds

Method

Cook the beets and roast them at 375 degrees F for an hour and allow to cool. Unpeel and chop into half inch cubes. In a medium sized skillet over high heat, onion, vinegar, broth, sugar, and orange peel and bring to a boil, stirring often, until liquid is reduced to tbsp., about 5 minutes. Mix pomegranate seeds into the beet combination and salt to flavor. Serve without delay.

Enjoy!

Delicious Corn and Black Bean Salad

Ingredients

1 tbsp. plus 3 tbsp. olive oil

1/2 onion, chopped

1 cup corn kernels, from about 2 ears of corn

12 tbsp. chopped cilantro

1 15 1/2-oz. can black beans, drained and rinsed

1½ tomatoes, about 0.5 lbs., cored, seeded and chopped

1½ tbsp. red wine vinegar

1 tsp. Dijon mustard

Salt and pepper

Method

Keep your oven to preheat to 400 degrees F. Place 1 tbsp. oil in an ovenproof skillet and heat on high. Sauté the onions until tender. Add in the corn kernels and keep stirring until soft. Place the skillet in the preheated oven and broil until the vegetables are brown, stirring often. This will take about 20 minutes. Immediately remove in a plate and allow to cool. Place the cooled corn mix in a bowl and add in the tomatoes, cilantro and beans and mix well. In a small bowl pour in the vinegar, mustard, pepper and salt and mix well until the salt dissolves. Slowly add in the 3 tbsp. oil and keep whisking until all the ingredients are well incorporated. Pour this dressing over the corn mix and serve immediately.

Enjoy!

Crispy Broccoli Slaw

Ingredients

4 slices bacon

1/2 large head broccoli

1/2 small red onion, minced, 1/2 cup

3 tbsp. golden raisins

3 tbsp. mayonnaise

1½ tbsp. white balsamic vinegar

2 tbsp. honey

Salt and pepper

Method

Brown the bacon slices in a skillet until crisp. Drain it on a kitchen towel and crumble it into half inch pieces. Keep aside. Separate the florets from the broccoli and chop the stem into bite sized pieces. Place in a large bowl and mix together with the raisins and onion. In another bowl combine the vinegar and mayonnaise and mix until smooth. Pour in the honey and season with salt and pepper. Just before serving pour the dressing over the broccoli mix and toss to coat. Top with the crumbled bacon and serve immediately.

Enjoy!

Bistro-Style Salad

Ingredients

1 ½ tbsp. finely chopped walnuts

2 large eggs

Cooking spray

1 bacon slice, uncooked

4 cups gourmet salad greens

2 tbsp., 0.5 ounce crumbled blue cheese

1/2 Bartlett pear, cored and thinly sliced

½ tbsp. white wine vinegar

1/2 tbsp. extra virgin olive oil

1/4 tsp. dried tarragon

1/4 tsp. Dijon mustard

2, 1-inch-thick slices French bread baguette, toasted

Method

Roast the walnuts in a small skillet until an aroma fills the kitchen. This should take about 3-4 minutes when cooking on high heat. Remove and keep aside. Spray 2 6 ounce custard cups with the cooking spray. Break an egg in each custard cup. Using a plastic wrap cover them both and microwave on high for 40 seconds or until the eggs are set. Set aside for 1 minute and remove on a paper towel. Brown the bacon in a skillet until crisp. Drain and crumble. Reserve the fat. In a large bowl mix together the crumbled bacon, roasted walnuts, salad greens, blue cheese and pear. In another small bowl combine about 1 tsp. of fat, vinegar, oil, tarragon and mustard and whisk until combined. Just before serving drizzle the dressing over the salad and serve topped with the egg and French baguette on the side.

Enjoy!

Spinach and Blackberry Salad

Ingredients

3 cups Baby spinach, washed and drained from the water

1 pint Fresh blackberries

1 pint Cherry tomatoes

1 sliced Green onion

¼ cup finely chopped walnuts

6 ounces Crumbled feta cheese

½ cup Edible flowers

Bacon dressing or balsamic vinegar as per choice

Method

Mix baby spinach, blackberries, cherry tomatoes, green onions, walnuts together by tossing them together. Add cheese and toss again. This salad tastes good; with or without any salad dressing. If you want to add a dressing, use bacon dressing or plenty amount of balsamic vinegar as per your choice. Before serving, top with any edible flower you like.

Enjoy!

Vegetable Salad with Swiss Cheese

Ingredients

1 cup Green onions, sliced

1 cup Celery, sliced

1 cup Green pepper

1 cup Pimiento-stuffed olives

6 cup Shredded lettuce

1/3 cup Vegetable oil

2 cup Shredded Swiss cheese

2 tbsp. Red wine vinegar

1 tbsp. Dijon mustard

Salt & pepper to taste

Method

Combine the olives, onions, celery, and green pepper in a salad bowl and toss well. Whisk together the oil, mustard, vinegar in a small bowl. Season the dressing with salt and pepper. Sprinkle the dressing over the vegetables. Refrigerate overnight or several hours. Before serving, line the plate with lettuce leaves. Mix cheese with the vegetables. Place the salad on the lettuce. Top it with shredded cheese. Serve immediately.

Enjoy!

Tasty Carrot Salad

Ingredients

2 pounds Carrots, peeled and cut into thin diagonal slices

½ cup Flake of almonds

1/3 cup Dried cranberries

2 cups Arugula

2 cloves of Garlic minced

1 packet Crumbled Danish blue cheese

1 tbsp. Cider vinegar

¼ cup Extra-virgin olive oil

1 tsp. Honey

1-2 pinch Freshly grounded black pepper

Salt to taste

Method

Combine the carrots, garlic, and almonds in a bowl. Add a little olive oil and mix it well. Add salt and pepper to taste. Transfer the mixture to a baking sheet and bake in the preheated oven for 30 minutes at 400 degrees F or 200 degrees C. Take them out when the edge turns brown and allow them to cool. Transfer the carrot mix in a bowl. Add honey, vinegar, cranberries and cheese and toss well. Mix arugula and serve immediately.

Enjoy!

Marinated Vegetable Salad

Ingredients

1 can tiny green peas, drained

1 can French-style green beans, drained

1 can White or shoe peg corn, drained

1 medium Onion, thinly sliced

¾ cup finely chopped celery

2 tbsp. Chopped pimientos

½ cup White wine vinegar

½ cup Vegetable oil

¾ cup Sugar

½ tsp. Pepper½ tsp. Salt

Method

Take a large bowl and combine peas, corns and beans. Add celery, onion and pimientos and toss the mixture well. Take a saucepan. Put all the remaining ingredients and cook on low flame. Stir continuously till the sugar gets dissolved. Pour the sauce over the vegetable mixture. Cover the bowl with a lid and refrigerate overnight. You can keep it for several days in the refrigerator. Serve chilled.

Enjoy!

Roasted Colorful Corn Salad

Ingredients

8 Fresh corn in husks1 Red Bell pepper, diced

1 Green bell pepper, diced

1 red Onion, chopped

1 cup Chopped fresh cilantro

½ cup Olive oil

4 cloves of Garlic, crushed then minced

3 Limes

1 tsp. White sugar

Salt & pepper to taste

1 tbsp. hot sauce

Method

Take a large pot and place the corn in it. Pour in water and soak the corn for 15 minutes. Remove the silks from the husks of the corn and keep aside. Take a griller and preheat it at high temperature. Place the corn over the grill and cook for 20 minutes. Turn them occasionally. Allow to cool and discard the husks. Take a blender and pour the olive oil, lime juice, hot sauce in it and give it a whirl. Add in the cilantro, garlic, sugar, salt, and pepper. Blend to form a smooth mixture. Drizzle over the corn. Serve immediately.

Enjoy!

Creamy Cucumber

Ingredients

3 Cucumbers, peeled and thinly sliced

1 Onion, sliced

2 cups Water

¾ cup Heavy whipping cream

¼ cup Cider vinegar

Minced fresh parsley, optional

¼ cup Sugar

½ tsp. Salt

Method

Add water and salt the cucumber and onions, allow to soak for at least 1 hour. Drain excess water. Whisk together the cream and vinegar in a bowl until smooth. Add the marinated cucumbers and onion. Mix well to coat evenly. Refrigerate for few hours. Before serving, sprinkle parsley.

Enjoy!

Marinated Mushroom and Tomato Salad

Ingredients

12 ounces Cherry tomatoes, halved

1 package Fresh mushrooms

2 sliced green Onions

¼ cup Balsamic vinegar

1/3 cup Vegetable oil

1 ½ tsp. White sugar

½ tsp. Ground black pepper

½ tsp. Salt

½ cup Chopped fresh basil

Method

In a bowl, whisk the balsamic vinegar, oil, pepper, salt and sugar to form a homogenous mixture. Take another large bowl and mix the tomatoes, onions, mushrooms, and basil together. Toss well. Add the dressing and evenly coat the vegetables. Cover the bowl and refrigerate 3-5 hours. Serve chilled.

Enjoy!

Bean Salad

Ingredients

1 can Kidney beans, washed and drained

1 can Garbanzo beans or chickpeas, washed and drained

1 can Green beans

1 can Wax beans, drained

¼ cup Julienne from green pepper

8 green Onions, sliced

½ cup Cider vinegar

¼ cup Canola oil

¾ cup Sugar

½ tsp. Salt

Method

Combine the beans together in a large bowl. Add the green pepper and onions to the beans. In a covered jar whisk the cider vinegar, sugar, oil, and salt to form smooth dressing. Let the sugar completely dissolve in the dressing. Drizzle over the bean mixture and toss well. Cover the mixture and refrigerate overnight.

Enjoy!

Beet Salad with Garlic

Ingredients

6 Beets, boiled, peeled and sliced

3 tbsp. Olive oil

2 tbsp. Red wine vinegar

2 cloves of Garlic

Salt to taste

Green onion slices, few for garnish

Method

Combine all the ingredients in a bowl and toss well. Serve immediately.

Enjoy!

Marinated Corn

Ingredients

1 cup Frozen corn

2 green Onions, thinly sliced

1 tbsp. Chopped green pepper

1 Leaf lettuce, optional

¼ cup Mayonnaise

2 tbsp. Lemon juice

¾ tsp. Ground mustard

¼ tsp. Sugar

1-2 pinch Freshly grounded pepper

Method

Mix the mayonnaise with the lemon juice, mustard powder, and sugar together in a large bowl. Whip it well until smooth. Add corn, green pepper, onions, to the mayonnaise. Season the mixture with salt and pepper. Cover and chill it in the refrigerator overnight or at least 4-5 hours. Before serving, line the plate with lettuce and place the salad over it.

Enjoy!

Pea Salad

Ingredients

8 slices Bacon

1 packet Frozen green peas, thawed and drained

½ cup chopped Celery

½ cup chopped Green onions

2/3 cup Sour cream

1 cup Chopped cashews

Salt and pepper to taste

Method

Put bacon in a large pan and cook it over medium or medium high flame till both the sides get browned. Drain extra oil with a paper towel and crumble the bacon. Keep it aside. Mix celery, peas, scallions and sour cream together in a medium sized bowl. Toss well with a gentle hand. Add cashews and bacon into the salad just before serving. Serve immediately.

Enjoy!

Turnip Salad

Ingredients

¼ cup Sweet red pepper, chopped

4 cups Shredded peeled turnips

¼ cup Green onions

¼ cup Mayonnaise

1 tbsp. Vinegar

2 tbsp. Sugar

¼ tsp. Pepper

¼ tsp. Salt

Method

Take a bowl. Mix red pepper, onions and toss. Take another bowl for preparing the dressing. Mix mayonnaise, vinegar, sugar, salt and pepper and whisk it well. Pour the mixture over the vegetable and toss well. Take turnips in a bowl add this mixture to the turnip and mix well. Refrigerate the vegetable overnight or for several hours. More marinating will incorporate more taste. Serve chilled.

Enjoy!

Apple and Avocado Salad

Ingredients

1 packet Baby greens

¼ cup Red onions, chopped

½ cup Chopped walnuts

1/3 cup Crumbled blue cheese

2 tsp. Lemon zest

1 Apple, peeled, cored and sliced

1 Avocado, peeled, pitted and diced

4 Mandarin oranges, juiced

½ Lemon, juiced

1 clove of Garlic minced

2 tbsp. Olive oil Salt to taste

Method

Mix the baby greens, walnuts, red onions, blue cheese, and lemon zest together in a bowl. Toss the mixture well. Whisk vigorously the mandarin orange juice, lemon zest, lemon juice, minced garlic, olive oil. Season the mixture with salt. Pour over the salad and mix. Add the apple and avocado to the bowl and toss just before serving the salad.

Enjoy!

Corn, Bean, Onion Salad

Ingredients

1 can whole kernel corn, washed and drained

1 can tiny peas wash and drained

1 can Green beans, drained

1 jar Pimientos, drained

1 cup Finely chopped celery

1 Onion, finely chopped

1 Green pepper, finely chopped

1 cup Sugar

½ cup Cider vinegar

½ cup Canola oil

1 tsp. Salt

½ tsp. Pepper

Method

Take a large salad bowl and combine the onion, green pepper, celery together. Keep it aside. Take a sauce pan and pour the vinegar, oil, sugar, salt and pepper and bring it to a boil. Remove from heat and allow the mixture to cool. Drizzle over the vegetables and toss well to evenly coat the veggies. Refrigerate several hours or overnight. Served chilled.

Enjoy!

Italian veggie Salad

Ingredients

1 can Artichoke hearts, drained and quartered

5 cups Romaine lettuce, rinsed, dried, and chopped

1 Red bell pepper, cut into strips

1 Carrot1 Red onion, thinly sliced

¼ cup Black olives

¼ cup Green olives

½ Cucumber

2 tbsp. Grated Romano cheese

1 tsp. Chopped fresh thyme

½ cup Canola oil

1/3 cup Tarragon vinegar

1 tbsp. White sugar

½ tsp. Dry mustard

2 cloves of Garlic minced

Method

Take a medium container with tight lid. Pour canola oil, vinegar, dry mustard, sugar, thyme, and garlic. Cover the container and whisk vigorously to form a smooth mixture. Transfer the mixture to a bowl and place artichoke hearts in it. Refrigerate and let it marinate overnight. Take a large bowl and combine the lettuce, carrot, red bell pepper, red onion, olive, cucumber, and cheese together. Toss gently. Add salt and pepper to season. Mix it with the artichokes. Allow to marinade for four hours. Serve chilled.

Enjoy!

Seafood Pasta Salad

Ingredients

1 package tricolor pasta

3 stalks celery

1 pound imitation crabmeat

1 cup frozen green peas

1 cup mayonnaise

½ tbsp. white sugar

2 tbsp. white vinegar

3 tbsp. milk

1 tsp. salt

¼ tsp. ground black pepper

Method

Boil a large pot of salted water, add pasta and cook for 10 minutes. When pasta is boiling, add the green peas and crabmeat. In a large bowl, mix the other mentioned ingredients and keep aside for some time. Mix in the peas, crabmeat and pasta. Serve immediately.

Enjoy!

Grilled Vegetable Salad

Ingredients

1 pound trimmed fresh asparagus

2 zucchini, halved lengthwise and end are trimmed

2 yellow squash

1 large sliced red onion

2 red bell peppers, halved and seeded.

½ cup extra virgin olive oil

¼ cup red wine vinegar

1 tbsp. Dijon mustard

1 clove minced garlic

Salt and ground black pepper to taste

Method

Heat and grill the vegetables for 15 minutes and then remove vegetables from grill and chop them into small pieces. Add other ingredients and toss the salad so that all the spices are well mixed. Serve immediately.

Enjoy!

Delicious summer corn salad

Ingredients

6 ears husked and totally cleaned corn

3 large chopped tomatoes

1 large chopped onion

¼ cup chopped fresh basil

¼ cup olive oil

2 tbsp. white vinegar

Salt and pepper

Method

Take a large pot, put water and salt and boil it. Cook corn in that boil water then add all the ingredients listed. Toss the mixture well and refrigerate. Serve chilled.

Enjoy!!

Crunchy Pea Salad with caramel

Ingredients

8 slices bacon

1 package dried frozen green peas

½ cup chopped celery

½ cup chopped green onions

2/3 cup sour cream

1 cup chopped cashews

Salt and pepper according to your taste

Method

Cook bacon in a pan over medium heat until browned. Mix the other ingredients, except for the cashews in a bowl. Finally add bacon and cashews over the mixture. Toss well and serve immediately.

Enjoy!

Black Bean Magic Salad

Ingredients

1 can rinsed and drained black beans

2 dried cans of kernel corn

8 chopped green onions

2 seeded and minced jalapeno peppers

1 chopped green bell pepper

1 peeled, pitted and diced avocado.

1 jar pimentos

3 seeded and chopped tomatoes

1 cup chopped fresh cilantro

1 lime juiced

½ cup Italian salad dressing

½ tsp. garlic salt

Method

Take a large bowl and put all ingredients in it. Toss it well so that they mix well. Serve immediately.

Enjoy!

Yummy Greek Salad

Ingredients

3 large ripe chopped tomatoes

2 peeled and chopped cucumbers

1 small chopped red onion

¼ cup olive oil

4 tsp. lemon juice

½ tsp. dried oregano

Salt and pepper according to taste

1 cup crumbled feta cheese

6 black Greek olives, pitted and sliced

Method

Take a medium sized bowl and mix the tomatoes, cucumber and onion very well and leave that mixture for five minutes. Sprinkle oil, lemon juice, oregano, salt, pepper, feta cheese and olives over the mixture. Toss and serve immediately.

Enjoy!!

Amazing Thai Cucumber salad

Ingredients

3 large peeled cucumbers that must cut into ¼ inch slices and seeds are to be removed

1 tbsp. salt

½ cup white sugar

½ cup rice wine vinegar

2 jalapeno chopped peppers

¼ cup chopped cilantro

½ cup chopped peanuts

Method

Combine all the ingredients in a large mixing bowl and toss well. Season according to taste and serve chilled.

Enjoy!

High protein tomato basil salad

Ingredients

4 large ripe sliced tomatoes

1 pound fresh mozzarella sliced cheese

1/3 cup fresh basil

3 tbsp. extra-virgin olive oil

Fine sea salt

Fresh ground black pepper

Method

On a plate alternate and overlap tomato and mozzarella slices. Finally put some sprinkle of olive oil, fine sea salt and pepper over it. Serve fresh, topped with the basil leaves.

Enjoy!

Quick Cucumber Avocado salad

Ingredients

2 medium cubed cucumbers

2 cubed avocado

4 tbsp. chopped fresh cilantro

1 clove minced garlic

2 tbsp. chopped green onion

¼ tsp. salt

Black pepper

¼ large lemon

1 lime

Method

Take the cucumbers, avocado and cilantro mix them well. Finally add pepper, lemon, lime, onion and garlic. Toss it well. Serve immediately.

Enjoy!

Mouth Watering Orzo and Tomato Salad with Feta Cheese

Ingredients

1 cup uncooked orzo pasta

¼ cup pitted green olives

1 cup diced feta cheese

3 tbsp. chopped fresh Presley

1 ripe chopped tomato

¼ cup virgin olive oil

¼ cup lemon juice

Salt and pepper

Method

Cook orzo according to the manufacturer's instructions. Take a bowl and mix the orzo, olives, parsley, dill and tomato very well. Finally put salt, pepper and on top add feta cheese. Serve immediately.

Enjoy!

English Cucumber and Tomato Salad

Ingredients

8 Roma or plum tomatoes

1 English cucumber, peeled and cubed

1 cup Jicama, peeled and thinly chopped

1 small Yellow bell pepper

½ cup Red onion, cubed

3 tbsp. Lemon juice

3 tbsp. extra virgin olive oil

1 tbsp. Dried parsley

1-2 pinch of Pepper

Method

Combine together the tomatoes, bell pepper, cucumber, jicama, and red onion in a bowl. Toss well. Pour olive oil, lemon juice and coat the mixture. Sprinkle the parsley and toss. Season it with salt and pepper. Serve immediately or chilled.

Enjoy!

Grandma's Eggplant Salad

Ingredients

1 Eggplant

4 Tomatoes, cubed

3 Eggs, hard-boiled, cubed

1 Onion, thinly chopped

½ cup French salad dressing

½ tsp. Pepper

Salt, for seasoning, optional

Method

Wash eggplant and cut it half lengthwise. Take a baking dish and grease it with olive oil. Arrange the eggplants cut side down in the greased baking dish. Bake for 30-40 minutes at 350 degrees F. Take it out and allow to cool. Peel the eggplant. Cut them into small cubes. Take a large bowl and transfer the eggplant to it. Add onion, tomatoes, eggs, dressing, pepper and salt. Toss well. Freeze at least 1 hour in the refrigerator and serve.

Enjoy!

Carrot, Bacon and Broccoli Salad

Ingredients

2 heads Fresh broccoli, chopped

½ pound Bacon

1 bunch Green onions, chopped

½ cup Shredded carrots

½ cup Raisins, optional

1 cup Mayonnaise

½ cup Distilled white vinegar

1-2 pinch Pepper

Salt to taste

Method

Cook bacon in a large, deep pan over medium high flame until brown. Drain and crumble. Combine the broccoli, green onions, carrots and bacon in a large bowl. Add salt and pepper. Toss properly. Take a small container or bowl and put the mayonnaise and vinegar and whisk. Transfer the dressing to the vegetable mixture. Coat the vegetables with a gentle hand.

Refrigerate at least 1 hour and serve.

Enjoy!

Cucumber and Tomato Salad with Sour Cream

Ingredients

3-4 Cucumbers, peeled and cut slices

2 Lettuce leaves, for decoration, optional

5-7 Slices of tomatoes,

1 Onion, thinly sliced into rings

1 tbsp. Minced chives

½ cup Sour cream

2 tbsp. White vinegar

½ tsp. Dill seed

¼ tsp. Pepper

Pinch of sugar

1 tsp. Salt

Method

Place the cucumber slices in a bowl and sprinkle salt. Marinate for 3-4 hours in the refrigerator. Take out the cucumber and wash. Drain all the liquid and transfer in a large salad bowl. Add onion and keep aside. Take a small bowl and combine vinegar, sour cream, chives, dill seed, pepper and sugar in it. Whisk the mixture and pour it over the cucumber mixture. Toss gently. Arrange the plate nicely with lettuce and tomato. Serve immediately.

Enjoy!

Tomato Flavored Tortellini Salad

Ingredients

1 pound Rainbow tortellini pasta

3 Plum tomatoes cut into halves

3 ounces Hard salami, diced

2/3 cup Sliced celery

¼ cup Sliced black olives

½ cup Red bell pepper

1 tbsp. Red onion, diced

1 tbsp. Tomato paste

1 clove of Garlic minced

3 tbsp. Red wine vinegar

3 tbsp. Balsamic vinegar

2 tsp. Dijon mustard

1 tsp. Honey

1/3 cup Olive oil

1/3 cup Vegetable oil

¾ cup Shredded provolone cheese

¼ cup Chopped fresh parsley

1 tsp. Chopped fresh rosemary

1 tbsp. Lemon juice

Pepper & salt to taste

Method

Cook pasta according to the instructions on the packet. Pour cold water and drain. Keep it aside. Using a broiler, broil the tomatoes until the skin becomes partially blackened. Now process tomato in the blender. Add the tomato paste, vinegars, garlic, honey and mustard and blend again. Gradually add olive oil and vegetable oil and blend until smooth. Add salt and pepper. Combine pasta with all the vegetables, herbs, salami, and lemon juice in a bowl. Pour the dressing and toss well. Serve.

Enjoy!

Broccoli and Bacon in Mayonnaise Dressing

Ingredients

1 bunch Broccoli, cut into florets

½ small Red onion, finely chopped

1 cup Shredded mozzarella cheese

8 Bacon strips, cooked and crumbled

½ cup Mayonnaise

1 tbsp. White wine vinegar

¼ cup Sugar

Method

Put broccoli, cooked bacon, onion, and cheese in a large salad bowl. Toss with a gentle hand. Cover and set it aside. Mix mayonnaise, vinegar and sugar in a small container. Whisk continuously till the sugar melts and forms a smooth mixture. Pour the dressing over the broccoli mix and coat evenly. Serve immediately.

Enjoy!

Chicken Salad with Cucumber Cream

Ingredients

2 cans Chicken chunks, drained from its juice

1 cup Seedless green grapes cut into halves

½ cup Chopped pecans or almonds

½ cup Chopped celery

1 can Mandarin oranges, drained

¾ cup Creamy cucumber salad dressing

Method

Take a large, deep salad bowl. Transfer the chicken, celery, grapes, oranges and pecans or almond as per your choice. Toss gently. Add cucumber salad dressing. Coat the chicken and vegetable mixture evenly with the creamy dressing. Serve immediately.

Enjoy!

Vegetables with Horseradish Dressing

Ingredients

¾ cup Cauliflower florets

¼ cup Cucumber

¼ cup Chopped seeded tomato

2 tbsp. Sliced radishes

1 tbsp. Sliced green onions

2 tbsp. Diced celery

¼ cup Cubed American cheese

For Dressing:

2 tbsp. Mayonnaise

1-2 tbsp. Sugar

1 tbsp. Prepared horseradish

1/8 tsp. Pepper

¼ tsp. Salt

Method

Mix the cauliflower, cucumber, tomato, celery, radish, green onion, and cheese together in a large bowl. Keep it aside. Take a small bowl. Mix mayonnaise, sugar, horseradish until the sugar melt and forms a smooth mixture. Pour the dressing over the vegetables and toss well. Refrigerate for 1-2 hours. Serve chilled.

Enjoy!

Sweet Pea and Pasta Salad

Ingredients

1 cup Macaroni

2 cups Frozen green peas

3 Eggs

3 green Onions, chopped

2 stalks Celery, chopped

¼ cup Ranch salad dressing

1 tsp. White sugar

2 tsp. White wine vinegar

2 Sweet pickles

1 cup Shredded cheddar cheese

¼ Freshly grounded black pepper

Method

Cook pasta in the boiling water. Add a pinch of salt in it. When done, rinse it with cold water and drain. Take a saucepan and fill it with cold water. Add eggs and bring it to a boil. Remove from flame and cover. Let the eggs stand in warm water for 10-15 minutes. Take the eggs out of warm water and allow to cool. Peel the skin and chop. Take a small bowl and combine salad dressing, vinegar, and sugar. Whisk well and season with salt and freshly grounded black pepper. Combine the pasta, eggs, vegetables and cheese. Pour dressing and toss. Serve chilled.

Enjoy!

Colorful Pepper Salad

Ingredients

1 Green pepper, julienned

1 Sweet yellow pepper, julienned

1 Sweet red pepper, julienned

1 Purple pepper, julienned

1 Red onion, julienned

1/3 cup Vinegar

¼ cup Canola oil

1 tbsp. Sugar

1 tbsp. Minced fresh basil

¼ tsp. Salt

Dash of pepper

Method

Take a large bowl and combine all the peppers and toss it well. Add onion and toss again. Take another bowl and combine the remaining ingredients and whisk the mixture vigorously. Drizzle the dressing over the pepper and onion mixture. Toss nicely to coat the veggies. Cover the mixture and put it in the refrigerator overnight. Serve chilled.

Enjoy!

Chicken, Sun-Dried Tomato and Pinenut Salad with Cheese

Ingredients

1 loaf of Italian bread, cubed

8 Grilled chicken strips

½ cup Pine nuts

1 cup Sun-dried tomatoes

4 green onions cut into 1/2-inch pieces

2 packages mixed salad greens

3 tbsp. extra virgin olive oil

½ tsp. Salt

½ tsp. freshly ground black pepper

1 tsp. Garlic powder

8 ounces feta cheese, crumbled

1 cup Balsamic vinaigrette

Method

Mix the Italian bread and olive oil. Season it with salt, garlic powder, and salt. Put the mixture in a single layer in the greased 9x13 inch baking dish. Place it in the preheated broiler and broil until it turns brown and toasted. Take it out and allow to cool. In a baking sheet line the pine nuts and place it in the bottom rack of the broiler oven and toast carefully. In a small bowl, take hot water and soak sun-dried tomatoes in it until soft. Slice the tomatoes. In a salad bowl, mix all the green veggies; add tomatoes, pine nuts, croutons, grilled chicken, vinaigrette and cheese. Toss well. Serve.

Enjoy!

Mozzarella and Tomato Salad

Ingredients

¼ cup Red wine vinegar

1 clove Garlic minced

2/3 cup Olive oil

1 pint Cherry tomatoes halved

1 ½ cups Cubed part-skim mozzarella cheese

¼ cup Chopped onion

3 tbsp. Minced fresh basil

Pepper to taste

½ tsp. Salt

Method

Take a small sized bowl. Add vinegar, minced garlic, salt and pepper and mix until the salt dissolves. Add the oil and whisk the mixture until smooth. In a large bowl, add tomatoes, cheese, onion, basil and mix it with a gentle hand. Add the dressing and toss well. Cover the bowl and put it in the refrigerator for 1 to 2 hours. Stir occasionally. Serve chilled.

Enjoy!

Spicy Zucchini Salad

Ingredients

1 ½ tbsp. Sesame seeds

¼ cup Chicken broth

3 tbsp. Miso paste

2 tbsp. Soy sauce

1 tbsp. Rice vinegar

1 tbsp. Lime juice

½ tsp. Thai chili sauce

2 tsp. Brown sugar

½ cup Chopped green onions

¼ cup Chopped cilantro

6 Zucchini, julienned

2 sheets Nori cut into thin slices

2 tbsp. Slivered almonds

Method

Put sesame seeds in a pan and place over the medium flame. Cook for 5 minutes. Stir continuously. Toast it lightly. Combine the chicken broth, soy sauce, miso paste, rice vinegar, lime juice, brown sugar, chili sauce, green onions, and cilantro together in a bowl and whisk. In a large salad bowl, toss the zucchini and the dressing to coat evenly. Top the zucchini with toasted sesame seeds, almonds and nori. Serve immediately.

Enjoy!

Tomato and Asparagus Salad

Ingredients

1 pound Fresh asparagus, cut into 1-inch pieces

4 Tomatoes, cut into wedges

3 cups Fresh mushrooms, sliced

1 Green pepper, julienned

¼ cup Vegetable oil

2 tbsp. Cider vinegar

1 clove Garlic minced

1 tsp. Dried tarragon

¼ tsp. Hot pepper sauce

¾ tsp. Salt

¼ tsp. Pepper

Method

In a pan, take a small amount of water and cook asparagus in it till becomes crisp and tender, nearly about 4-5 minutes. Drain and keep it aside. In a large salad bowl, combine the mushrooms with tomatoes, and green pepper. Combine other remaining ingredients in another bowl. Combine the vegetable mixture with the dressing. Toss well and cover and keep in the refrigerator for 2 to 3 hours. Serve.

Enjoy!

Minty Cucumber, Onion and Tomato Salad

Ingredients

2 Cucumbers, halved lengthwise, de-seeded and sliced

2/3 cups coarsely chopped red onion

3 Tomatoes, de-seeded and coarsely chopped

½ cup Chopped fresh mint leaves

1/3 cup Red wine vinegar

1 tbsp. granulated no calorie sweetener

1 tsp. Salt

3 tbsp. Olive oil

A dash of pepper

Salt to taste

Method

Combine together the cucumbers, granulated sweetener, vinegar, and salt in a large bowl. Allow it to soak. It should be left at room temperature for at least 1 hour to marinate. Occasionally, stir the mixture. Put the tomatoes, onion, chopped fresh mint to it. Toss well. Add oil to the cucumber mixture. Toss to coat evenly. Add salt and pepper according to taste. Serve chilled.

Enjoy!

Adas Salatas

(Turkish lentil salad)

Ingredients:

2 cups Lentils, cleaned

4 cups Water

¼ cup Olive oil

1 Onion, sliced

2-3 cloves Garlic, sliced

2 tsp. Ground cumin

1-2 Lemons, juice only

1 bunch Parsley, sliced

Salt and boost to taste

2 Tomatoes, cut into wedges (optional)

2 Eggs, hard-boiled and cut into wedges (optional)

Black olives, optional

¼ cup Feta milk items, optional , crumbled or sliced

Method

Add the beans and water to a huge pot and boil over medium-high fire. Decrease the heat, secure and prepare until ready through. Do not overcook. Drain and wash with cold water. Heat the olive oil in a sauté pan over medium heat. Add the red onion and sauté until just clear. Add the garlic cloves and cumin and sauté for another 1 or 2 minutes. Place the beans in a huge dish and add the red onion, tomatoes and eggs. Mix in the lemon juice, parsley, boost and salt. Serve fresh topped with the cheese.

Enjoy!

Ajvar

Ingredients:

3 Medium eggplants, cut in half, lengthwise

6-8 Red sweet peppers

½ cup Olive oil

3 tbsp. Vinegar or clean fresh loaded orange juice

2-3 cloves Garlic, sliced

Salt and boost to taste

Method

Preheat the oven to 475 degrees F. Put the eggplant cut-side down on a carefully oiled baking sheet and cook until the styles are blackened and the eggplant is ready through, about 20 minutes. Remove to a huge dish and cover to steam for a few minutes. Place the sweet peppers on the baking sheet and cook in the oven, flipping, until the skin is blackened and the sweet peppers are soft, another 20 minutes or so. Remove to another dish and cover to steam for a few minutes. After the clean vegetables have chilled, remove the pulp of the eggplant into a huge dish or a mixer, eliminating the rest of the parts. Cut the sweet peppers and add them to the eggplant. Use a spud masher to mash the eggplant and sweet peppers together until smooth, but still a little coarse. If using a mixer, beat the combination to the desire structure instead. Stir in the remaining elements and season to taste.

Enjoy!

Bakdoonsiyyeh

Ingredients:

2 bunches Italian parsley, sliced

¾ cup Tahini

¼ cup Lemon juice

Salt to taste

Water

Method

Whisk together the tahini, clean fresh loaded orange juice and salt in a mixing bowl until smooth. Add a tbsp. or two of water as required to make a dense dressing. Season to taste. Add the sliced parsley and toss. Serve immediately.

Enjoy!

Causa Rellena

Ingredients:

2 pounds Yellow, Yukon gold celery

½ cup Oil

¼ cup Lime or clean fresh loaded orange juice

2-3 amarillo chili place, optional

Salt and boost to taste

2 cups Filling

2-3 Hard-boiled egg, sliced

6-8 Pitted black olives

Method:

Place the celery in a huge pot of salted water. Heat to a boil and cook the celery until they are soft and ready through. Keep aside. Put the celery through a ricer or mash with a spud masher until smooth. Mix in the oil, boost (if using), calcium mineral or clean fresh loaded orange juice and salt to taste. Line a lasagna pan dish. Distribute 50 % the celery into the bottom of the dish and smooth out. Distribute the preferred stuffing similarly over the celery. Distribute the remaining celery similarly over the stuffing. Lay an offering dish upside-down over the top of the causa dish. Using both hands, turn the dish and dish over, enabling the causa fall onto the dish. Garnish the causa decoratively with the hard-boiled egg and olives and, if you like, a spices. Cut into sections and provide.

Enjoy!

Curtido

Ingredients:

½ head Cabbage

1 Carrot, peeled and grated

1 cup beans

4 cups Boiling water

3 sliced Scallions

½ cup White apple cider vinegar

½ cup Water

1 Jalapeno or serrano chili boost

½ tsp. Salt

Method

Place the vegetables and beans in a huge heat-proof dish. Add the sizzling water into the dish to cover the vegetables and beans and set aside for about 5 minutes. Drain in a colander, forcing out as much fluid as possible. Return the vegetables and beans to the dish and toss with the remaining of the elements. Let set in refrigerator for a couple hours. Serve chilled.

Enjoy!

Gado Gado

Ingredients

1 cup Green Gram beans, boiled

2 Carrots, peeled and sliced

1 cup Green beans, cut into 2-inch measures, steamed

2 Potato, peeled, boiled and sliced

2 cups Romaine lettuce

1 Cucumbers, peeled, cut in rings

2-3 Tomatoes, cut into wedges

2-3 egg hard boiled, cut into wedges

10-12 Krupuk , shrimp crackers

Peanut Sauce

Method

Combine all the ingredients, except for the romaine lettuce, and mix well.

Serve the salad on a bed of the romaine lettuce.

Enjoy!

Hobak Namul

Ingredients

3 Hobak or zucchini crush, cut into half moons

2-3 cloves Garlic, chopped

1 tsp. Sugar

Salt

3 tbsp. Soy marinade

2 tbsp. Toasted sesame oil

Method

Bring a pot of water to a steam over medium-high fire. Add the crush, and cook for about 1 minute. Drain and wash with cold water. Drain again. Mix together all the ingredients and mix well. Serve warm with a selection of Japanese sides and a main meal.

Enjoy!

Horiatiki Salata

Ingredients

3-4 Tomatoes, seeded and chopped

1 Cucumber, peeled, seeded and chopped

1 Red onion, sliced

½ cup Kalamata olives

½ cup Feta cheese, chopped or crumbled

½ cup Olive oil

¼ cup apple cider vinegar

1-2 cloves Garlic, chopped

1 tsp. Oregano

Salt and spice up to taste

Method

Toss the fresh vegetables, olives and dairy products together in a huge, non-reactive plate. In another plate, mix together the olive oil, apple cider vinegar, garlic cloves, oregano, spice up and add salt. Pour the dressing into the plate with the fresh vegetables and mix. Set aside to marinate for half an hour and serve it warm.

Enjoy!

Kartoffelsalat

(German spud salad)

Ingredients

2 pounds apples

¾ cup hot meat or poultry soup

1 Onion, chopped

1/3 cup Oil

¼ cup Vinegar

2 tbsp. Brown or Dijon mustard

1 tbsp. Sugar

Salt and spice up to taste

1-2 tbsp. Chives or parsley, chopped, optional

Method

Place the apples into a huge pot and add enough water to cover them by inches or two. Place over medium-high warm and bring to a boil. Decrease heat to low, and continue to steam until the apples are prepared through and a knife pierces them easily. Strain and set aside to cool. Cut the apples into quarters. Combine all the ingredients together and mix well. Adjust the dish to taste and serve warm, at 70 degrees for the best taste.

Enjoy!

Kvashenaya Kapusta Provansal

Ingredients

2 pounds Sauerkraut

1 Apple, cored and chopped

1-2 Carrot, peeled and grated

4-6 Scallions, chopped

1-2 tbsp. Sugar

½ cup Olive oil

Method

Add all the ingredients in a large bowl and mix well. Adjust seasoning as per taste and serve chilled.

Enjoy!

Waldorf Chicken Salad

Ingredients:

Salt and pepper

4, 6- to 8-ounce boneless, skin free poultry breasts, no more than 1 inches wide heavy, trimmed

½ cup mayonnaise

2 tbsp. lemon juice

1 tsp. Dijon mustard

½ tsp. ground fennel seeds

2 celery rib cage, minced

1 shallot, minced

1 Granny Smith peeled, cored, cut in half, and cut into ¼-inch pieces

1/2 cup nuts, chopped

1 tbsp. sliced fresh tarragon

1 tsp. sliced fresh thyme

Method

Dissolve 2 tbsp. salt in 6 cups cold water in a pot. Immerse poultry in water. Heat the pot over warm water until 170 degree Celsius. Turn off the heat and let it stand for 15 minutes. Return the poultry to paper towel–lined plate. Refrigerate until poultry is chilled, about half an hour. While the poultry cools, mix mayonnaise, lemon juice, mustard, ground fennel, and ¼ tsp. boost together in large plate. Pat poultry dry with sponges and cut into ½-inch pieces. Return poultry to plate with mayonnaise mixture. Add oatmeal, shallot, the apple juice, nuts, tarragon, and thyme; toss to mix. Season with the boost and add salt to taste. Serve.

Enjoy!

Lentil Salad with Olives, Excellent, and Feta

Ingredients:

1 cup beans, picked over and rinsed

Salt and pepper

6 cups water

2 cups low-sodium poultry broth

5 garlic cloves, lightly crushed and peeled

1 bay leaf

5 tbsp. extra-virgin olive oil

3 tbsp. white wine vinegar

½ cup coarsely sliced rough Kalamata olives

½ cup fresh great outcomes in, chopped

1 large minced shallot

¼ cup crumbled feta cheese

Method

Soak the beans in 4 cups of hot water with 1 tsp. of salt in it. Drain well. In a saucepan combine the beans, remaining water, broth, garlic, bay leaves and salt and cook until the beans soften. Drain and discard the garlic and bay leaves. In a bowl, combine with rest of the ingredients and mix well. Serve topped with some feta cheese.

Enjoy!

Thai Grilled-Beef Salad

Ingredients:

1 tsp. paprika

1 tsp. capsicum spice up pepper

1 tbsp. white rice

3 tbsp. calcium mineral juice, 2 limes

2 tbsp. fish sauce

2 tbsp. water

½ tsp. sugar

1, 1 ½ pound flank meal, trimmed

Salt and white boost, coarsely ground

4 shallots, sliced thin

1 ½ cups fresh great outcomes in, torn

1 ½ cups fresh cilantro leaves

1 Thai Chile, stemmed and sliced thin into rounds

1 seedless English cucumber, sliced 1/4 inches wide heavy on bias

Method

Grill the flank meals on high heat until medium rare. Keep aside to rest. Slice into bite sized pieces. In a bowl combine all the ingredients and toss well until mixed. Serve immediately.

Enjoy!

All-American Salad

Ingredients

1 little head red cabbage, shredded

1 large carrot, grated

1 apple, cored and chopped

Juice from, at least 50 % a Key lime

25 white seedless grapes, sliced

1/2 cup nuts, chopped

3/4 cup raisins, golden raisins look best, but I prefer regular for taste

1/2 white onion, chopped

4 tbsp. mayonnaise

Method

In the order listed, add all the elements to a large plate. Stir well after adding lime juice to all the contents.

Enjoy!

CPSIA information can be obtained
at www.ICGtesting.com
Printed in the USA
LVHW081520100222
710600LV00011B/335

9 781804 500064